Facial Rejuvenation

Acupressure

Look 10 Years Younger
In 10 min Per Day

Anne Cossé

Facial Rejuvenation Acupressure

Look 10 Years Younger
In 10 min Per Day

Onze Heures Huit

Facial Rejuvenation Acupressure
An Onze Heures Huit Publishing book
May 2008

For information address:
www.annecosse.com

Cataloging-in-Publication Data:
(National Library Board, Legal Deposit Office, Singapore 486548)
Cossé, Anne
The Facial Rejuvenation Acupressure Guide
ISBN 978-2-9527960-2-6

The information contained in this book is intended to be educational and not for diagnosis, prescription, or treatment of any health disorder whatsoever. This information should not replace consultation with a competent healthcare professional. The content of this book is intended to be used as an adjunct to a rational and responsible healthcare program prescribed by a healthcare practitioner.
The author and publisher are in no way liable for any misuse of the material.

Photographer: Vincent Cossé

Contents

Facial Rejuvenation Acupressure:
the Natural Rejuvenating Beauty Treatment

Beauty is a generic word that encompasses so many factors. This program aims at helping you looking your best *you*. More precisely: fresh, radiant, plump.

Why Exercise Your Face?

Aging

Over time, our metabolism slows down and does not work as well as in our youth. It doesn't produce enough collagen, doesn't keep moist as well, cells renew at a slower pace, etc. Our face looks dryer, duller, more tired, less plump, the skin wrinkles.

Acupressure can slow down the slowing down of our metabolism, if you will, and therefore the wrinkling, dehydration, dullness of complexion.

Gravity

Age is not the only culprit. Gravity as well progressively takes its toll on the human body, especially the face.

Gravity keeps pulling muscles, skin, and tissues downwards. Over the years, the connective tissue (the substance attaching the skin to the muscles) weakens, causing the skin to slip down, away from the muscles. The results are wrinkles and sags.

When you exercise your face, you strengthen the bond between the skin and muscles, improving tone and facial countours.

Health

As they say, "beauty comes from within". Looking good is not just a matter of facial traits. It stems from how we feel, interact and handle stress. All these elements contribute to a fresher, younger look.

Stress and fatigue worsen frown lines, creases and wrinkles. They tend to tense and block certain areas and points on the face. By working on those points, we work on the root of the problem, and tension and its consequences can be alleviated.

What is Acupressure?

Acupressure is an ancient knowledge, originating in China 5,000 years ago. It is based on a complex approach of the human body, where all levels are intertwined: physical, emotional, mental and spiritual.

Eastern tradition describes the world in terms of energy. It is the elementary substance and vital force of life. All living beings have this energy. It goes way beyond simple muscular energy. It encompasses all the energies a body can pull: physical, mental, physiological and psychological. This flow bears different names on the planet: Qi or Ch'i in Chinese (as in Qi Gong and Tai Chi Chuan), Ki in Japanese (as in Aikido) and Prana in India. In the West, it is referred to as bio-electricity by the scientists, and orgone (by Dr W. Reich).

According to traditional Chinese medicine, the Qi is always moving, and is constantly fed by external sources (food and fluids intake, air, sun, relationships). It depends as well on our personal inherited potential.

The same way blood is transported by the veins system, vital energy circulates in the body along a net of subtle paths: the meridians. The meridians link the physical sphere to emotions and psyche. They are the key to a balanced and healthy state.
At some specific spots on the path, the Qi gets near the skin and is thus physically accessible. Those key spots are the famous acupuncture points, or acupoints. They are the gateways to the Qi, and to the whole energy system. To work on the acupoints, acupuncture uses needles, and acupressure uses gentle to firm finger pressure (and fist, elbow, feet, depending on the technique).

How Does Acupressure Work to Rejuvenate the Face?

Acupressure is a finger pressure technique. Therefore it can be used as a facial massage technique. Simple finger pressure relieves congested areas as well as relaxes the muscles. Thus toxins are released and eliminated, which of course benefits our outward appearance.

More importantly, many meridians run across the face, neck and skull. By massaging the points linked to the Qi, acupressure accesses the deeper levels and works on the general well-being, which in turn reflects on the face (everybody has noticed how a person in love looks radiant no matter what!). This vital energy is the most important element of Facial Rejuvenation Acupressure; it governs our health, how we feel as well as how we look.

Although acupressure is orignally a therpeutic art (a medicine), the Chinese have used it to enhance facial beauty for thousands of years. It shown effective for toning muscles, improving the condition and luster of skin. Some points are even named *Facial Beauty* and *Heavenly Appearance.*
Applied to facial beauty, acupressure becomes a powerful, non-invasive, natural tool to rejuvenation.

And the good news is: you can do it yourself, and all you need is... your hands!
No tool (except your fingers) or extensive and costly treatment programs are required. Once the exercises are learned, you can use them for the rest of your life!

Facial Rejuvenation Acupressure:
Guidelines & Suggestions

The skin on your face is delicate and fragile. Massaging in this area should be done with care. Furthermore, acupoints are in direct connection with your inner vital force, and there are a few recommendations to follow to enhance the effect of their stimulation, as for any acupressure session.

Get prepared
Before practicing any facial acupressure exercise, wash your hands in warm water. Remove your make-up. If your skin is dry, ightly moisturize it. Try to use organic soap and lotions.

Never pull your skin
During the exercises you will have to reposition your fingers from one point to another. To do so, do not drag the skin. First, release the pressure from the point you just worked. Then move your hand to reposition it to the next point.

Practice slowly
Acupressure is not more effective when we press harder or move faster. Better results are achieved by practicing in (very) slow motion. Pressure is to be applied gradually and consciously into each point. Facial muscles respond better that way.

Breathe deeply
To help you stay relaxed and aware, take slow, deep breathes all through the exercises. Deep breathing helps as well to regulate the metabolism, and that in turns enhances the benefits of the movements and pressure.

Practice in front of a mirror
If you find it difficult to find the points on your face, practice the facial exercises in front of a mirror. That technique is used by dancers when they practice. It helps gain greater control and confidence. At the beginning, watch yourself closely, then try to practice the exercises with your eyes closed. You will automatically concentrate on what you are doing and what you are feeling during the exercises.

Relax
You will enjoy the exercises more and get greater benefits if you practice in a state of deep relaxation. Whenever possible, practice in a comfortable, quiet, private environment. At work, a meeting room or even the toilets can be the solution!

After the exercises, take a few minutes to reconnect with the world. Stay still in a sitting position, close your eyes, don't forget to breathe deeper than usual. Rub the palms of your hands together briskly to create heat, and immediately place your hands lightly over your face. Feel the warmth and the gentle tingling on your eye lids. After a minute or so, let your hands rest on your lap, relax your arms and shoulders and slowly reconnect with your environment, until you can open your eyes and go.

Frequency and duration

Like for a diet, there are two phases to the process: once you achieve the results, you need a maintenance program. After you tone your facial muscles, you must continue the program to maintain the benefits.

Phase 1: Achieving the results

For the first 2 weeks or so (it depends on your own particular face), try to practice the daily routine twice a day. If you skip a session don't panic, it is still working. Just try to not skip the next session. For the next 2 weeks or so, practice the daily routine once a day only.

Note: During those weeks, gradually increase the time you practice the exercises. Start with approximately a half minute for each step, and gradually increase the time each week, slowly building to a minute.

The exact duration of time needed varies; it takes longer to fade the deep lines.

Phase 2: Maintaining the results

Once you achieve the results you wanted, continue the same routine three times a week as a maintenance program, or two times in relaxed periods (holidays, for instance).

The Complete Facial Rejuvenation Acupressure Program:
The Daily Eight Steps Routine

Start with a Smile

A big smile is also a great way to feel good!

Position the heels of your hands on the edge of your temples, at eyes level. Your palms and fingers rest naturally on the sides of your head.

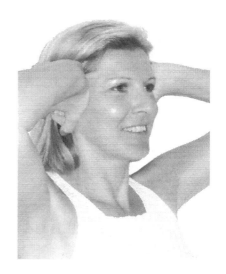

Smile
Slightly tilt your chin downward. Relax your mouth and let it open about one inch. Smile.

Breathe
Take five long deep breaths. Make sure your shoulders muscles stay relaxed. Let your arms rest in your lap, and your face relax.

1. UPPER PART OF THE FACE

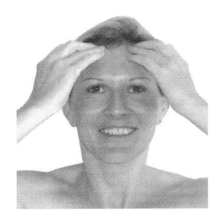

Hairline

With your fingertips find the crevices along your hairline. For some of us these indentations are hollow.

Every crevice is an acupressure point. Place the forefinger, middle and ring fingers of your right hands on the crevices located on the right side of your hairline. Do the same with your left hand

Close your eyes. Calm your mind. With your shoulders relaxed, apply direct firm pressure into these indentations. Take deep slow breaths. Reposition your fingertips into the next indentations and apply pressure.

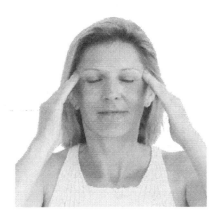

Temples

Place the cushion of your forefinger, middle and ring fingers fingertips on your temples, on both sides of your forehead.

The bone there is like a large, hollow, circular indentation. Fit your fingertips into this indentation.

Apply pressure and make a slow circular rotation. Go very slow, so as to gently stretch the skin in all directions without pulling too hard.

Eye Brows

Place your elbows on a table and your fingertips under the upper ridge of the eye socket. Let your head rest on your fingertips, so as to allow the weight of your head to do the job of applying pressure into the points. Breathe slowly and deeply, and make sure your arms and shoulders are relaxe.
Hold for a count of ten.
If the points are sore or just sensitive, apply lighter pressure and hold longer.

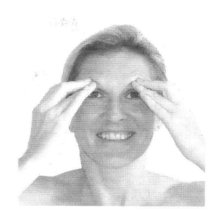

Lower Eye Ridge

Place your fingertips on the lower ridge of the eye socket. Find the point located on the edge (thickness) of the bone. You might need to push your fingertip a little bit in the orbit, so that the cushion sits on the edge of the ridge bone. Breathe slowly and deeply.

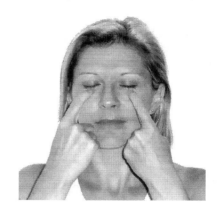

Frown lines

Find the crevices that sit all across your forehead. They form a lline above the inner corner of the eye, a lline above the pupil and a line above the outer corner of the eye. Beware: the illustration shows symetry, but in real life we are not perfectly symetrical.

Place the fingertip of your ring finger on point #1, middle finger on point #2 and forefinger on point #3. Apply pressure by rolling the fingertips from side to side. Then reposition your fingertips one point up until you worked the whole line. Repeat on the next line.
Then repeat on the other side.

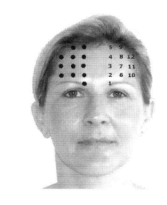

2. THE EYES

For this exercise, make sure your neck, shoulders and arms don't get tense, and that you breath slowly and deeply.

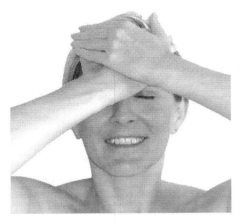

Pumping

Place the center of the palm of your right hand on the 3rd eye. This chakra, located between your eyebrows, is also an acupressure point. Cover your right hand with your left hand. Gently "pump" the heel in and out 10 times as you breathe deeply.

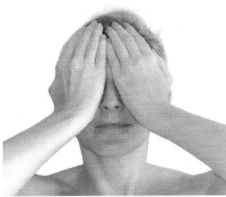

Palming

Form a slight C with your hands, and place the palms over your eyesockets. Rest the fingers on your forehead. Hold while breathing deeply and slowly. Be aware of what you feel (tingling, warmth, calm) and what you see (sparkles, colors, etc).

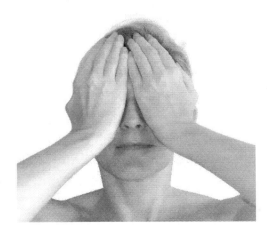

Resisting

Keep your palms in the same position. Press firmly the edge of your palms (not the center, that would press directly on your eyeballs) ont he bones where they sit.

Try to shut both eyes tightly while resisting the movement with the pressure of your cupped palms. Hold for 5 counts. Release and repeat 3 more times.

With the same cupping technique over your eyes, resist the movement under your hands while you make the following expressions:

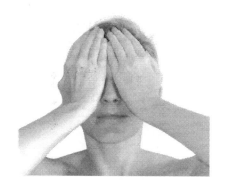

Frowning
Pull your eyebrows inwards, then lift your eyebrows straight up. Hold each position for 3 counts. Repeat twice.

Squinting
Make a big smile and squint your eyes. Hold for 3 counts and relax. Repeat twice.

Orbiting the Eyes
Place your thumbs under the upper ridge of your eyesocket so that the pads fit underneath the ridge (on the edge of the bone). Press firmly, yet slowly and gently. Start with the point located at the inner corner of the eye. Apply pressure, release. Reposition a bit more to the outer side, and repeat (press, release, reposition). Work your way to the outer edge of your eyesocket.

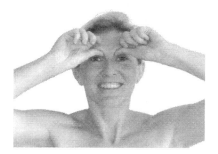

Use your forefinger and middle fingers to continue orbiting around on the lower ridge underneath the eye. Remember to lift your fingers off the skin before you reposition them, to avoid stetching and pulling the delicate skin in this area.

3. MIDDLE PART OF THE FACE

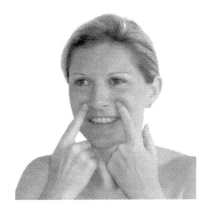

Nose

Place your forefingers on the edge of the nostrils, pressing up in towards the gravity center of your head. Breathe deeply and hold for a slow count of ten.

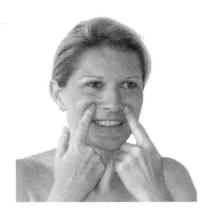

Cheekbones

Reposition your forefingers slightly outward and add your middle fingers. Press firmly across the base of your cheek bones toward your ears. Press the points underneath your cheekbone, pausing at the Facial Beauty point (on the cheekbone, at pupil level). Let your head rest on your fingertips so tha it's weight does the pressure work.
Repeat this 3 times.
Pause at the most sensitive points and hold them for 20 to 30 seconds.

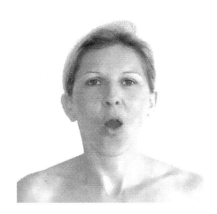

Mouth

Form a loose "O" with your lips. Tense your mouth muscles to form a smaller "O", and resist at the same time opening your mouth wide, for 10 counts.
Breathe deeply.
Repeat once for 10 counts.

4. LOWER PART OF THE FACE

This step tones the skin and muscles in the jawline, improving facial contour.

Jaw line

Form a hook with your forefinger, and position your thumb below, with the pad facing up.

Hook onto your jawline. Use the top knuckles of your forefinger to apply pressure into the top jawbone while the lower jaw rests on your thumb.

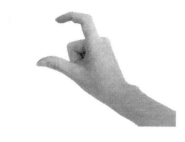

Start on the median line of your face (see picture), apply pressure, make small rotations with the knuckles of your forefinger, release, reposition outward and repeat across the jaw to your ears.

Make sure your thumbs are hooked firmly under the jawbone, so as to stimulate as well the points located in this area.

Repeat twice from the median line.

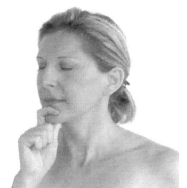

Chin

Press your tongue up against the roof of your mouth. Push as firmly as you can. Place the flat of your hand (knuckle side up) underneath the chin area, holding firmly to a count of 10. Release both the tongue and fingers.
Repeat once, but this time pat the underchin area briskly with your hand. Then hold for a count of 10.

Repeat this entire jawline exercise one more time.

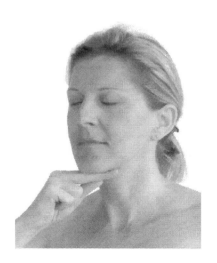

5. THE NECK

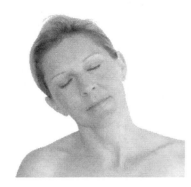

Inhale slowly and deeply. On the exhale, slowly tilt your head to one side, with your ear trying to touch your shoulder (without lifting the shoulder). Go slowly, especially if you experience any stiffness.
Inhale again while you bring your head back to an upright position.
Repeat on the other side.
Repeat this exercise twice, moving slowly from side to side in sync with your breathing.

Butterfly Neck Press

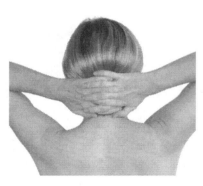

Interlace your fingers behind your neck. While inhaling deeply, lean your head back and bring your elbows out, stretching the chest area as open as you can. Hold for 3 counts.
Make sure your shoulders don't get tense.

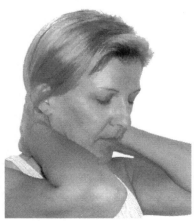

On the exhalation, slowly drop your head forward, and let your elbows move close to each other, even touching if you can. Hold for 3 counts.

Repeat 4 more times, inhaling up and exhaling down, to release any tension in your neck.

Again, make sure your shoulders and arms don't get tense in the process.

END WITH AN EARS RUB

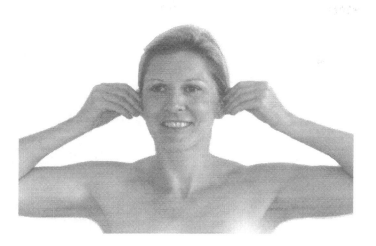

There are over 150 points on each ear that affect all parts of the body. Rubbing your ears is a delightful way to relax and energize your whole system at the same time!

Briskly rub your hands together to generate heat and electricity. Take hold of each ear and thoroughly massage the outer auricle with your thumb and forefinger as shown above. Continue down to the lobe area, but don't rush. Firmly knead your ears for several minutes, until they feel warm and vibrant.
End by holding them completely in your full hands and gently rolling them.

The Express Facial Rejuvenation Routine:
1 Minute to a Relaxed Glow

All the movements in this exercise have to be done consciously, in a very slow motion. Breathe deeply, and concentrate on what you are doing.

Skull

Cup both hands open, and run all your fingertips on your skull upwards from the ears, in a very slow motion. Start on the sides of the head up to the middle of the hairline. Repeat once. Find the occipital bump behind the ears, and run your fingertips upwards to the top of your skull. Repeat once. Start from the occipital ridge behind the head, and move upwards to the top of the skull. Repeat once. Massage any occipital bump you find.

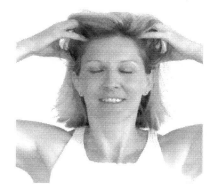

Forehead

Place the forefingers, middle and ring fingertips of both hands on the Third Eye. Run them vertically towards the middle of your hairline, as if you wanted to iron your forehead.
Place your fingertips on the middle of the upper eye ridge. Run them vertically towards the hairline.
Place your fingertips on your temples. Run them vertically towards the hairline.
Do not pull your skin. Just imagine you are ironing the muscles.

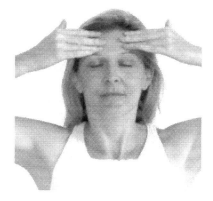

Cheekbones

Place your forefingertips at the base of your nose. Run them outwards, following the cheekbones. Repeat twice.

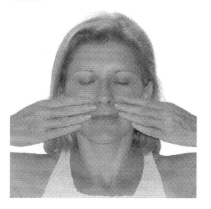

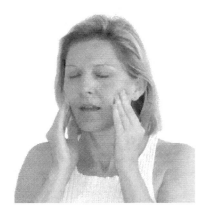

Jaws

Place all your fingertips on your jaw articulations. Relax your jaw by letting the lower jaw drop. Massage the muscles very slowly.

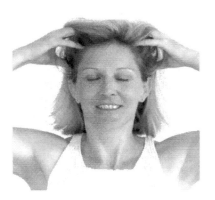

Skull

End this express routine by running the cushions of your fingertips along your skull, from the base of the occiput to the top of the head.

A La Carte Facial Rejuvenation

The two routines described earlier are complete programmes to apply regularly, be it for maintenance purpose.

There are other ways to use acupressure for facial beauty, and it is on specific areas, to alleviate specific conditions. Many meridians run across the face, neck and skull, and many key acupoints are located there. They can be worked on for a more focussed approach of beauty.

A facial area where aging takes visibly its toll is the eyes. The skin around the eyes is very thin and sensitive, and wrinkles are more obvious. Furthermore, a poor blood circulation, lack of sleep, and sometimes heredity generate dark circles. Finally, stress, bad sleep hygiene, and poor fluids draining generate puffiness that often times stay there. Acupressure is an efficient tool to prevent and reduce these conditions.

The nose and sinuses zones might become congested too, but less visibly than the eyes area. Nevertheless, such a congestion tampers with facial beauty and glow. This chapter will show you simple exercises to clear nasal congestion.

Tension, anxiety and stress commonly crystallise on neck and shoulders, stomach, and jaws. Progressively, jaws can become clenched, muscles hurt, and the whole face seems tense and severe. The Qi does not flow properly anymore, and the face does not radiate any positive glow. In periods of stress and tension, a quick exercise, as described further, is a true relief.

Depending on your needs, pick and choose the following exercises, and master your facial beauty!

Rejuvenating the Eyes

This exercise is based on the Taoist health system. It helps the blood flowing through, which prevents dark circles around the eyes. It also helps reducing pockets and congestion under the eyes.

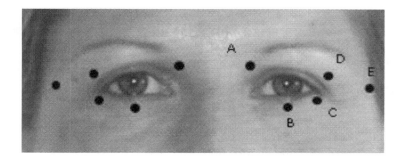

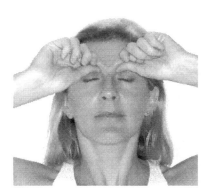

1. Position your thumbs in the indentation of the inner upper ridge of the eye sockets (A). Press firmly. It is often sore, which means those acupoints are blocked. If sore, release some pressure. Massage the points while counting to 10. Release.
Repeat 3 times.

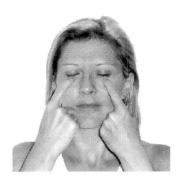

2. Position your forefingers in the indentations in the middle of the lower ridge of the eye sockets (B). Press firmly on the bone, not on the flesh. Massage the points while counting to 10. Release.
Repeat 3 times.

3. Move your forefingers to the outer corner of the lower ridge of the eye sockets (C). Press and massage the points while counting to 10. Release.
Repeat 3 times.

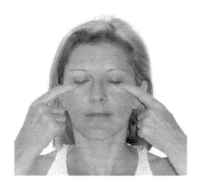

4. Position your middle fingers or thumbs to the outer corner of the upper ridge of the eye sockets (D). Press and massage the points while counting to 10. Release. Repeat 3 times.

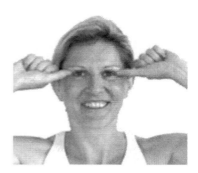

5. Place your middle fingers on your temples, in the indentation at the end of the eye brows (E). Press and massage the points while counting to 10. Release. Repeat 3 times.

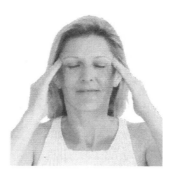

6. Briskly rub the palms of your hands together, until they feel very warm. Cover your eyes with your hands, your right hand partially covering your left hand if necessary. Do not press on the eyes. Count to 10. Repeat 3 times to feel the heat of your hands on your eyes.

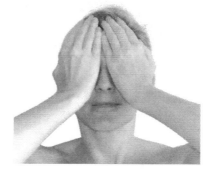

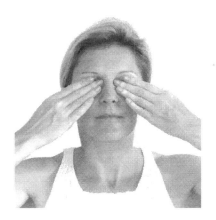

7. Lightly massage your eyes with your forefingers, middle, and ring fingers. Massage the bones around the eyes in a circular movement, starting with the inner corners close to the nose. Massage the nose bridge upwards, then along the eye brows to the temples, follow the lower ridge of the eyes to the nose. Repeat this movement 10 times. Release.
Repeat the cycle 3 times.

Notes:

- Always massage in the directions as indicated above, or you would weaken your eye muscles.
- If your eyes are congested, this exercise will release the stagnant lymph. Your vision might be blurred for a couple of minutes afterwards.
- Sore points do not need to be pressed on too firmly. In this case, light pressure is as efficient.
- Use an organic cream as lubricant, if necessary.

Decongestioning the Nose

This exercise is based on the Taoist health system. It helps reduce congestion along the nose, allowing fluids to drain out, and air to flow in.

With both your forefinger tips, press firmly on all the points as illustrated below.

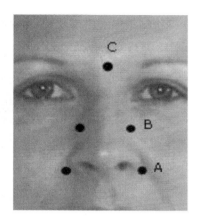

1. Start at the base of the nose, and press points (A) during 10 seconds. Then massage briefly.

2. Press the points located half way along the nose (B). Then massage briefly.

3. Press the point between the eye brows (the Third Eye) (C) with both fingers. Then massage briefly. Repeat routine 1-2-3 three times, always starting at the base of the nose, and finishing by the 3rd Eye.

4. Massage in a continuous movement, from the base of the nose to the points in the middle, to the Third Eye, to the middle of the forehead. Repeat this movement 3 times.

Notes:

- If in a hurry, do not accelerate the pace, but rather do the routine once only instead of three times. Try to use herbal cream.
- During the whole exercise, hold a deep and penetrating pressure. You might feel that some points are sensitive, or even sore. Soreness is due to blocage or emptiness in the meridian. Keep doing the exercise every day, and the pain will fade away. You will probably notice that you become less prone to sinusitis and allergies.

Unblocking the Sinuses

Symptoms of sinusitis are nasal congestion, headache, and pressure around the eyes and the bridge of the nose. These can cause muscular tension in the chest, which further blocks the sinuses.

Sinusitis have several possible causes.

1) If the fluids in the back of the nose are blocked and unable to drain, pressure builds up in the sinus areas. If this condition is not relieved, the swollen membranes inside the sinuses can eventually become infected.

2) The symptoms can be vaused by emotions, grief or fear. Using acupressure to release the tension might result is repressed emotions surfacing. Thos emotions can be dealt with directly, enabling the nasal passages of the sinuses to clear.

The acupressure point usually recommended to treat the sinuses is Large Intestine 4 (LI4), located at the intersection of the thumb and forefinger bones. LI4 is a decongestant point, that is why it can help to open up and drain the sinuses.

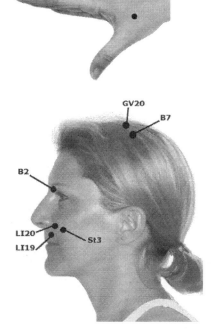

Other traditional acupressure points used to help open up the congested nasal passages are Governing Vessel 20 (GV20) and Bladder 7 (B7), located on the skull.

Bladder 2 (B2) is helpful for frontal headaches and sinus conditions. It is located at the bridge of the nose.

On the face, Large Intestine 19, 20 (LI19, LI20) and Stomach 3 (St3) are to be used for the maxillary sinuses. They are located in the cheek areas.

You might also want to try massaging the foot reflexology points associated with the sinuses: they are located on the sides and bottoms of the toes.

The Drilling Bamboo Exercise

This exercise helps working on the acupressure points mentioned above to relieve sinus problems.

Sit comfortably in a chair.

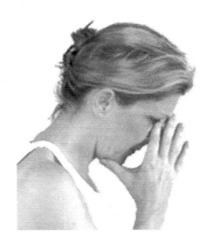

1. Position your forefingers on the points underneath the upper ridge of the eye socket, near the bridge of your nose (see B2 point).
Your middle finger will naturally rest near the Third Eye, located between the eye brows.
With your thumbs, hook your chin and hold that position for one minute.
Then move your thumbs to the hollow indentations of your temples for another minute.

2. Slowly inhale, lifting your head upward. Exhale as your head comes downward. Take long and deep breaths while you hold all the points.

3. With your fists, loosely pound or massage your chest muscles.

4. Place your hands on your lap. Sit straight and relax your shoulders (they should be downward). Close your eyes and deeply relax for another minute.

Relaxing the Jaws

Jaws are by excellence areas where tension crystallises, to the extent when it can even hurt.
Tension in the jaws can be generated by stress or because you grind your teeth when you are asleep. Overtime, tension and grinding can cause problems in the T.M.J. (temporal mandibular joint).

Locate the intersection between the upper and lower jaw.

With your middle fingers, apply prolonged, steady pressure directly on the muscle that pop out when you clench your teeth together. Hold this muscle for two minutes.

Then slowly move your jaws up and down, and side to side for an additional minute.
Release.

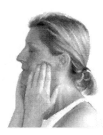

Dissolving a Headache

Headaches can be caused by dehydration or emotional stress. Your first action when your head aches should be to drink a big glass of water, and a second one an hour later. Often times, it fixes de problem.

However, some headaches are not that easy to get rid of. Emotions such as frustration, anger, worry and fear all put a strain on the shoulder, neck, and head muscles, causing pressures and tensions that can lead to headaches.

Tension tends to disturb the blood flow, and blood supplies oxygen. A headache is a signal of tension around the head, and there is a chance that your brain and face cells are not fed properly. And it shows.

The goal of the following exercise is to prevent such tension (which is a deeper relief than just taking a pill to relieve the symptoms).

The following routine can be done either lying down or sitting comfortably.

1. For one minute, use your fingertips to briskly rub all parts of your skull, as if you were shampooing your hair.

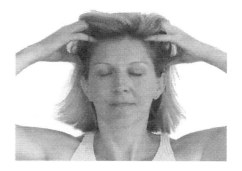

2. Then place your fingertips two inches directly above your belly button and gradually press into the pit of your stomach, while you breathe deeply for one minute.

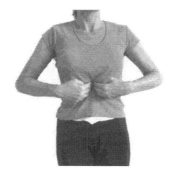

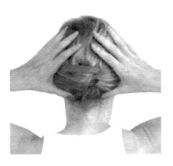

3. Use your thumbs to press underneath the base of your skull into the hollow areas on either side, two to three inches apart depending on the size of your head. Slowly tilt your head back with your eyes closed, and firmly press up underneath the skull for one or two minutes as you take long, deep breaths.

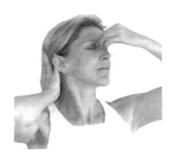

4. Use your right thumb to press the hollow spot at the base of your skull. Use your left thumb and forefinger to press the upper hollows of the eye socket near the bridge of the nose. Again, tilt your head back and breathe deeply for one or two minutes.

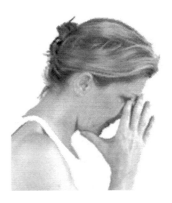

5. With the palms of your hands together, let your head tilt downward and position your forefingers and middle fingers on the Third Eye (between the eyebrows). Concentrate on this spot for two minutes as you breathe deeply.

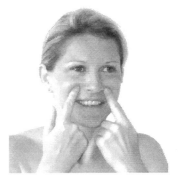

6. Use your forefinger of both hands to gently press up underneath the cheekbones, directly below the center of your eyes. Hold for one minute.

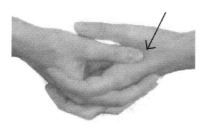

7. Place your right hand over the top of your left hand. Use your right thumb to press the webbing between the thumb and forefinger of your left hand. Angle the pressure toward the bone that connects with the forefinger. Hold for one minute. Then press this point for one minute on your opposite hand.

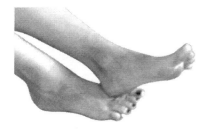

8. Slip off your shoes and sit down comfortably. Place your right heel on top of your left foot to rub in between the bones on the tops of your feet for one minute. Stimulate the sensitive spots between your big and second toes as well as between the bones that connect to your fourth and little toes. Then switch and work on the opposite foot.

Fighting Acne

Lifestyle is important. Indeed, an obvious way to get a clear complexion is to eat whole, natural foods and to get daily exercise (sweat cleans the skin and enables the pores to open).

However, regularly practicing facial rejuvenation acupressure exercises helps a lot. Here is why.

1) The routines increase blood and energy flows in the neck, face and skull.

2) When the bronchioles in the lungs become constricted due to stress and shallow breathing or congested from smoking, the condition is often externally reflected in the complexion. As a matter of fact, Traditional Chinese Medicine considers skin issues as an imbalance in the lungs and/or the large intestine meridians. The lungs meridian governs the skin, and specifically the pores. The pores enable the skin to breathe. Ten minutes of long, deep breathing exercises twice a day is an excellent way to prevent and manage acne and a dull complexion.

3) Refined, oily and rich foods leave waste materials in the colon. After a while they become toxic and block the colon (especially combined with a lack of exercise). Weakened intestines lead to constipation, and ultimately facial blemishes. The best preventive measure and remedy is a combination of exercise (which internally massages the colon) and a natural foods diet high in fiber.

4) Acne problems caused by a glandular imbalance might benefit from acupressure as well.

A good holistic health professional can help you to determine the source of the problem. In parallel, you can further improve your complexion with the following acupressure points.

Hoku Point: Firmly press the point in the webbing between your thumb and forefinger. Massage the Hoku point for one minute on each hand.

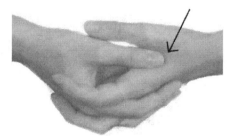

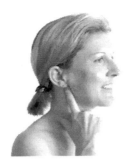

Heavenly Appearance Point:

That is the real name of acupressure point Small Intestine 17 (SI17). Beyond increasing the luster of the skin, this point also balances the thyroid gland and relieves hives.

It is located behind the jaw bone and a few inches below the ear lobe.
Lightly massage both in a gentle circular motion for one minute, twice a day.
Caution: the points can be sore, be gentle and do not overdo it.

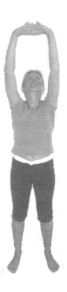

Breathing Exercise:
Stand up with your body relaxed.
Interlace your fingers together at your lap level.
Inhale as you raise your hands above your head, stretching your arms straight up. Tilt your head all the way back, looking upwards. Keep your neck muscles as relaxed as possible.
Separate your hands and exhale as you lower your hands down to your sides, shoulders down.
Repeat the exercise five more times, concentrating on breathing deeply and staying relaxed.

Glow & Lifestyle

The way we look depends on how we are and feel inside. You cannot glow if you feed your body with junk food, do not exercise, are ill or stressed out. If on the contrary you take care of your body and mind, it will show on your face.

Now that you know the facial rejuvenation acupressure points and how to work them, you can go one step further by improving your life style. When your whole body is healthy, it radiates energy, and you look beautiful. Athletes grind their body, musicians train their fingers, you can help your body better conveying and feeling the life force.

How To Set a Relaxing Environment

As simple and/or obvious as those suggestions might seem, we do not always think of them. Nonetheless, they are easy gestures, they do not cost much, and they make a big difference! Try at least two of them for a start, at home and in the office...

Clear out the clutter
It is difficult to feel centred when we are surrounded by unfinished business that constantly reminds us of what we haven't done yet. Ideally the only items on your desk/table/coffee table should be directly related to your current task/activity. Sort out the clutter daily, throw away what you do not need, and store (not shove) in an organized manner everything else in drawers, shelves, or cabinets.

Perfume the room
Light a scented candle, plug an air-freshener, use a Lampe Berger, put fragrant oil on the lamp bulbs, spray the air with home perfume, burn encense, add scented powder in your vacuum cleaner...
You can also be creative in your choice of scents: flowers and plants are diverse and pleasant, but some brands venture in the off-the beaten tracks with fragrances such as fire place, church, antique furniture wax, baking cake, chocolate... Explore.

Play soft music
Musical notes are vibrations, and as such resonate with our chakras. Choose music that suits your needs. Many relaxing music pieces are high-pitched and interact with the head chakras. Try also music with low bass vibrations, to interact with your lower chckras (groin to heart). It helps the mind to cool down, and the whole body to get grounded. Alternative stores have a wide offer, and can advise you.

Add plants
If you are blessed with green thumbs, use this gift! Even one plant makes a difference. An original place to try is the bedroom. Falling asleep below a tree is very relaxing.

Add a soothing decoration piece

If you find the sounds of running water soothing, consider adding a small fountain to your workspace, living room or bedroom. If you are visual, more than auditory, consider a mobile that moves gracefully with the breeze.

Set time for yourself

Negotiate a period of time each day where you turn off all outside communication, and encase yourself in a cocoon of concentration. Put up a "Do not disturb" sign at the door, turn off your phone, set your PC on sleep, ask your relatives/flatmates to stay away. Use this time to do what you please: read, stare at the ceiling, have a hot bubble bath, complete some red tape, write a season card, snooze, update your address book or schedule, try a new recipe, drink your favourite beverage...

How To Set a Healthy Life Style

Health care, called "Yang Sheng" in Chinese (literally: feed life), is essential in the ancient Chinese civilisation. It is based on an appropriate life style, including following simple Taoist diet principles. Like a Formula 1 engine, the human body needs the right fuel, oil, filters, etc to function in an optimal manner. What you eat is utterly important. And you have control on it.

The Qi can also be strengthened with health-oriented exercises such as Qi Gong and Tai Chi Chuan, traditional martial arts, or art forms such as the Tao Dance (Wutao).
The range of disciplines at your disposal is wide. This chapter develops some of them.

Diet

Nutrition is one of the pillars of traditional Chinese medicine, alongside herbal therapy, acupuncture, acupressure and Qi Gong. Nutrition is thus closely linked to our vital energy.

As an acupressure practitioner, although I do not give any diet instructions, I often observe a natural and progressive change in my patients' diet. Richard, for instance, a 63 year old senior who loves conviviality and excellent fare, wanted to get rid of his diabetes condition thanks to acupressure. His idea was that I would press a few points during a few sessions, and he would instantly slim down and reduce his cholesterol, while keeping eating a lot of heavy food... Instead of making him loose his illusions, and giving him dietary recommendations, which he would never have followed anyway, I underwent to rebalance his energy system, in a playful and convivial atmosphere. We would talk delicatessen, gastronomy recipes, and worthy restaurants. Not the usual appropriate speech!
After a few weeks of regular sessions, Richard started to raise all by himself an interest for broccolis (but cooked in a sexy way) and herbal tea (but carefully chosen spicy and virile by me), and is now rebalancing his diet. The acupressure work he receives has reawakened the link between him and his body. His body sends signals, and he hears them.

It is important to understand that *we become what we eat*. What we intake is transformed into our cells, our blood, our energy.

Chinese dietetics look at food energy, nature, savour, etc.
All nutrients are alive and have an energy, whether Yin or Yang. As a consequence, if we eat too much Yin food, our personality shifts to being more receptive, relaxed, nay passive. Eating only Yin food may weaken our organs.
Yang food, on the contrary, generates tightness and cohesion. An excess of Yang food brings more concentration, focus and structure to our personality. Our organs become harder, and may develop calculus (kidneys, gall bladder).

The ideal diet is a balance between Yin and Yang food, according to one's age, gender and lifestyle, and depending on the season.

Yang food ←------		------→ Yin food	
Hot, dry, nutritious, spicy. *Thickens the blood*		*Cold, humid, detoxifying.* *Dilutes the blood*	
Very Yang :	**Moderate Yang:**	**Moderate Yin:**	**Very Yin :**
Salt	Dry beans	Tofu	Exotic fruits
Poultry	Eggs	Local fruits	Citrus fruits
Fish	Algae	Nuts	Sugar
Meat	Root vegetable	Vegetable, sprouts	Alcohol
Wheat	Tubers	Dairy	Chemical products
Fried	Slightly sautéed	Steamed	Boiled
Tempura	Oven baked	Raw	Juice
Sautéed		Pressure-steam	

During summer: eat cold Yin food, fruits and green vegetables
During winter: eat more Yang food to warm yourself, beans and peas, root vegetables, and very few fruits.

As a rule of thumb, it is better to eat energy-filled food rather than dead or non natural food.

It is recommended to decrease or stop the intake of the following foods:
- Genetically modified
- Mass-produced
- Processed
- Industrial canned
- Unidentified transformed
- Non domestic
- Too Yin
- Too Yang

and prefer the following ones:

- Additive-free organic
- Hand-produced
- Non processed, whole
- Untransformed
- Local and regional
- Naturally preserved
- Wild

Alcohol, drugs

Alcohol and drugs unleash behaviour and personality. A few drinks, a marijuana cigarette, and one feels on top of the world: euphoric mood, apprehension gone, confidence boosted, sharpened senses, higher performance...

However, psychotropic substances do more than expanding one's conscience: they project it out of one's body. Alcohol throws the soul out of the liver (its natural nest, according to the Ancient eastern tradition), leaving space for toxic energies. Ecstasy, LSD and mushrooms cause dissociation between body and mind...

Furthermore, those substances have disastrous impacts on the vital energy: for instance, marijuana tarnishes the ethereal bodies, cocaine tears the aura...
Psychotropic substances, as well as being illegal, are dangerous for mental and physical health, and they get in the way of a natural beauty.

Tobacco

Nicotine is a substance that appears to stimulate the same brain zones as cocaine. Babies born from women smoking 6 to 7 cigarettes per day during their pregnancy present behavioural changes (excitement, tension, crying) similar to the new-born from women who absorbed crack, cocaine or heroin during their pregnancy (study from the Brown Medical School - USA).
Besides, smokers consume more tobacco when in situation of having to perform.
In parallel (and paradoxically), smoking a cigarette is relaxing. In fact, it soothes the artificial edginess generated by the physiological withdrawal of nicotine. In association with alcohol and drugs, tobacco is often used to relax. In fact, although this substance does not alter the conscience, it has all the other effects of psychotropic drugs.

Unfortunately, smoke and tar clog the lungs, the primary receptacle of the surrounding vital energy we breathe. Lungs are the main instruments of breathing, which is the technique on which all energy practices are based.
In addition, smoke lays down a grey veil on the ethereal bodies.
A clogged respiratory system is not an efficient tool for the fluidity of the energy in the body.

Environment

The vital energy is in us (Qi), but it is also in everything that surrounds us: the atmosphere, the ground, all other living creatures, nature. The quality of the air we breathe is essential, because air brings us more than oxygen: it brings some Qi. Thus, pollution is not a favourable environment for our energetic state, and beauty.

The trees and the sea are vital energy reservoirs. Walking in nature, touching and embracing a tree, gardening, put us in direct contact with the Ki, and we can fill ourselves with it. Walking on the beach, bathing in the sea, any activity that involves a contact with the sea at a maximum of 3 foot distance is a pleasant and efficient way to soak in Qi.
All the more if the air is pure!

Notes

Facial Acupressure Points Chart

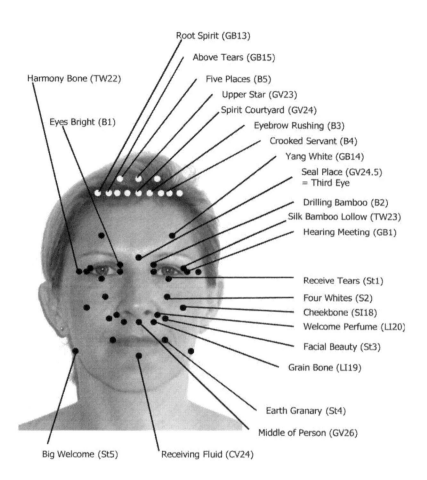

Root Spirit (GB13)
Above Tears (GB15)
Harmony Bone (TW22)
Five Places (B5)
Upper Star (GV23)
Spirit Courtyard (GV24)
Eyes Bright (B1)
Eyebrow Rushing (B3)
Crooked Servant (B4)
Yang White (GB14)
Seal Place (GV24.5)
= Third Eye
Drilling Bamboo (B2)
Silk Bamboo Lollow (TW23)
Hearing Meeting (GB1)
Receive Tears (St1)
Four Whites (S2)
Cheekbone (SI18)
Welcome Perfume (LI20)
Facial Beauty (St3)
Grain Bone (LI19)
Earth Granary (St4)
Middle of Person (GV26)
Big Welcome (St5)
Receiving Fluid (CV24)

Appendix

Points to avoid on pregnant women

Points whose stimulation sends the vital energy in the lower body, acts on the uterus or the fetus, or strengthens the Yang energy, should not be punctured on a pregnant woman. In addition, do not press heavily on the shoulders.

Three Miles (Stomach 36)
On the outer side of the leg (both right and left legs), 4 finger widths below the knee cap.

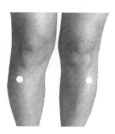

Adjoining Valley (Large Intestine 4)
In the webbing between the thumb and index finger.

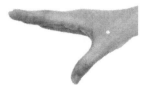

Three Yin Crossing (Spleen 6)
On the inner side of the lower leg, four finger-widths above the anklebone. The point is next to the back of the shinbone.

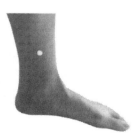

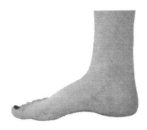

Big Stream (Kidney 3)

On the outer side of the ankle, in the depression behind the prominent ankle bone. The point is in the hollow between the tip of your ankle bone and the Achilles tendon, on the inner side of the ankle.

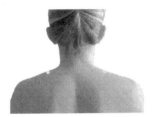

Shoulder Well (Gall Bladder 21)
On top of both shoulders, on the thick roll of muscle.
You will find the point midway between the outer tip of the shoulder and the base of the neck.

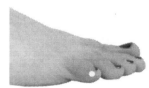

Reaching Inside (Bladder 67)
On the outside of the little toe, at the base of the toe nail.

About the author

Hi I am **Anne Cossé**.

I am a Certified Acupressure Practitioner by the State of California.

I am trained in traditional Shiatsu, Zen Shiatsu, Jin Shin Do, Reflexology, Touch for Health, and I am a Reiki Master & Teacher. To know more about me, visit www.annecosse.com

Since 2005 I have practiced therapeutic acupressure in Asia and Europe and delivered self-help acupressure workshops to thousands of people.
One of my thrills is to have been interviewed by many media around the world!

•

**For more TUTORIALS and more TIPS,
visit my blogs & social media:**

www.acupressurewellness.com

www.facialacupressure.com

www.youtube.com/annecosse

www.facebook.com/FacialRejuvenationAcupressure

https://plus.google.com/+annecosse

www.pinterest.com/annecosse

•

By the same author:

In English:

« Facial Rejuvenation Acupressure, the Complete Program
Look 10 Years Younger in 10 Min Per Day »
www.facialacupressure.com

« Boost your Weight Loss with Acupressure»
www.acupressurewellness.com

« Embrace Menopause, Natural Relief with Acupressure»
www.acupressurewellness.com

In French:

« Mon Massage Facial Anti-âge, Raffermir et Rajeunir en 10 Min par Jour »
www.rajeunirvisage.com

« Eliminer Poches et Cernes, Retendre et Lisser le Front »
www.rajeunirvisage.com

« Déclencher Mon Accouchement Naturellement avec l'Acupression »
www.declencheraccouchement.com

In Spanish:

« Rejuvenecimiento Facial, Belleza Natural en 10 Min por Dia »
www.amazon.es/Rejuvenecimiento-Digitopuntura-Fortalecer-Rejuvenecer-Minutos-
ebook/dp/B00AZO8IY6

Made in the USA
San Bernardino, CA
12 February 2020

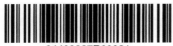